Taking Care of
Your Body

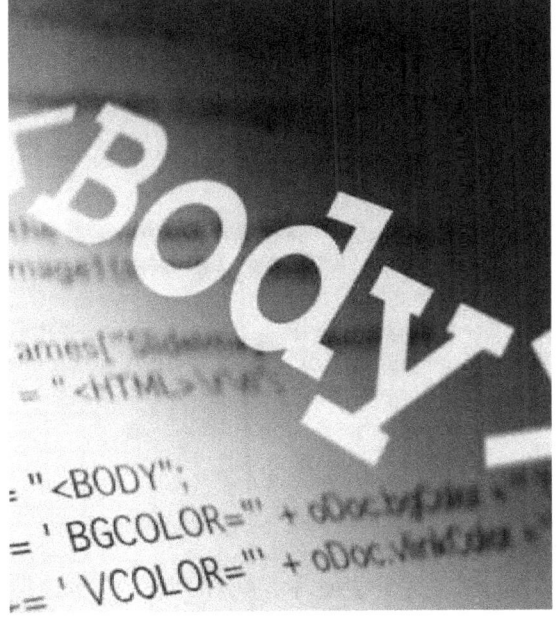

"Losing Weight At The Same Time"

By
Rita Knott-Woodfin

Title: Taking Care Of Your Body
Subtitle: *"Losing Weight At The Same Time"*
Copyright 2003 by Rita Knott-Woodfin

ISBN-13: 978-1500721176
ISBN-10: 1500721174

Vision Keepers Publication
P. O. Box 8212
Ranch Cucamonga, California 91701
951.318.3910

Printed in the United States of America

Disclaimer

The information contained in this book is not intended to diagnose or prescribe treatment, but is designed for educational use to promote health and wellness in every aspect of your life. The author, publisher, and/or distributor suggest you contact your physician prior to using the information contained in this book.

Table of Contents

About the Author............................ 7

Introduction................................... 9

Chapter 1   *Taking Care Of Your Body,*
             You Only Have One................13
Chapter 2   *Let's Get Started....................19*
Chapter 3   *Live a Longer and Healthier Life.....23*
Chapter 4   *The Positive Weight Loss Approach......27*
Chapter 5   *Where Diets Go Wrong................. 31*
Chapter 6   *Broth and Salad Recipes............. 35*
Chapter 7   *Vegetable and Fruit Juice Combinations..43*
Chapter 8   *Daily Schedule......................53*

Acknowledgments...........................59
Important Information............................61
Contact Information 63

About the Author

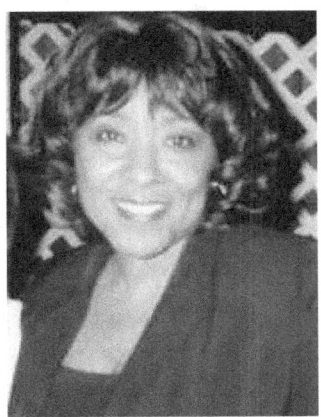

Rita Knott-Woodfin was born and raised in Tishabee, Alabama in the 50s and 60s, where food was the go to comforter for all ills, and the starter of lasting friendships. She learned early in life to always start the day with a full meal, and subsequently grew up cooking large meals for a large number of people on a daily basis. Therefore, early in life, she developed a passion for the "appetite" and extreme eating.

After moving to California at the age of eighteen and establishing a career soon after her arrival, she formed many lasting friendships -- most of which were formed around work, church, and of course, food.

After confessing Jesus Christ as her Savior and Lord 1n 1981, she was ordained as a minister in 1990 after serving the Lord in her local church for nearly ten years. She has been committed to the ministry for over 33 years. She is Founder/CEO of Vision Keepers Ministries, International. She has been ministering to broken women around the

Southern California area since 1989. As a motivational/inspirational speaker, she has encouraged the lives of thousands of women and men who otherwise would have lost hope, even for life itself.

Rita is the mother of three children and three grandchildren, which includes twin boys. She still has a strong passion for cooking and eating – which has brought her to this point in her life.

Her greatest desire is to make a positive impact on the life of each person she meets and to share the love of Jesus Christ with as many people as possible as she journeys through this life.

Introduction

Other than my love for God through Jesus Christ, food is my passion (yes, I said *it*). Even after the success of changing my way of eating thereby, changing my lifestyle, I must confess, I still have a passionate appetite. I love food! The difference is, I now know which foods to love.

My passion for food (eating) caused me to reach a level of weight that I never imagined. For the past twenty years of my life I slowly ate my way to a whopping 186 pounds (14 pounds from 200). Bear in mind that I am a woman of 5 feet 5 inches tall with a medium frame, and youth is not on my side.

At first I told myself that I was not over weight, but was only experiencing what comes with age. You know, "the metabolism slows down," "your body is getting ready for menopause," "weight gain is to be expected at your age," etc., etc. Well, I knew that I had to make some changes in my life or I was headed for some serious health problems, for sure. I did not perceive the 186 pounds as 186 pounds – I looked at it as "14 pounds from 200".

I began to experience constant tiredness, puffiness in my face, around my eyes, and in my feet and hands. I had every ache and pain you can think of. I felt lousy most of the time. I was getting up in the mornings feeling as if I had not gone to bed at all. I knew that I had to make changes in my diet as well as increasing my physical activity.

After joining gym after gym, paying the dues, and never attending; after many failed attempts to lose weight by trying diet after diet, that produced no results, I began to *PRAY* for answers.

I was desperate and determined to get my life back, lose weight, improve my quality of life; and get on the road to recovery and good health.

I asked the Lord for "HELP" and He gave me just that. Through a course of events, and in a very short period of time, the Lord led me to a very dear friend who had recently been diagnosed with diabetes. Because of her diagnoses she had taken drastic measures and changed her diet. This led to immediate weight loss and dramatically enhanced her health.

I began to try her way of eating. Then, with additional research, and much to my surprise, I was on to something that was about to change my life, forever. I purchased health and nutrition books to continue my research on a broader scale and from my findings I began to follow the recommendations.

In this book I will share with you some of my discoveries and successes and my desperation and commitment to change.

I began this program in the midst of the HOLIDAYS (Thanksgiving, Christmas, and New Year's). I was committed to make the change and was not going to delay it another day.

I also purchased the *"Colon Cleanse and Fiber Herbs," "Ultimate Cleanse by Nature's Way"* which was highly recommended to me during my research. I began to lose an average of "one half to one pound a day." Within one month of beginning this program, I had lost 29 pounds and had the energy of a *two year old!* *Imagine that...*

Those who knew me when, were shocked at what they saw. I have shared this information with many people. It has been mailed to people as far away as Germany.

I am so grateful for the success the Lord has given me, it is my desire that everyone who comes in contact with this information will make the commitment to obtain the same kind of success.

I don't remember ever feeling this energized and alive. Come, join me in an adventure to change!

God Bless

Rita Knott-Woodfin

Chapter 1

Taking Care Of Your Body,
You Only Have One

Are you feeling tired, run down, overweight, unable to do little more than get through the day with minimal activity?

Then the information in this book is just for "YOU."

How would you like to gain maximum spiritual awareness, great health, increased energy, mental clarity/alertness and lose weight at the same time? That's right! You can see a marked change in your spiritual and physical health, and lose weight at the same time, in a very short period of time – at the rate of approximately a pound a day. Sounds unreal? It's real and it's true. It has been proven time after time. Learn how to live as long as God as planned for you to live "The Healthy Way."

It's time to enjoy the health that God has in store for you. NO MORE EXCUSS. We have to ask ourselves, how did I get here, and how long did it take? The answer is, we have over-indulged by eating improperly and eating foods that can only enhance weight gain and cause our health to fail.

It's all in the foods and in the combinations of foods that we eat that cause bowel congestion and other mental and physical illnesses that plague us day in and day out.

What many of us have perceived to be a problem with our weight is really a problem with our ELIMINATION. This is called CONGESTED BOWELS. What we don't know is that nearly half of the entire human race is afflicted with constipation and other waste matter that is left in the body/colon entirely too long.

For most people, undigested food remains in the intestines from two weeks to three months, and even as long as a year. The longer the waste is retained in the intestines; the more poisons are being absorbed into the blood-stream.

It has been proven by medical authorities that nearly half of all diseases/sicknesses begin in the colon.

The liver, gall bladder, kidneys and other organs must all try to filter the excessive waste that is absorbed into the blood from the colon. When the colon is kept clean, disease in the body is very rare. However, when the bowels are sluggish, disease soon follows with the weakening of the immune system. Before trying to improve or cure any body ailment, the bowels must be in good working order.

The following information will teach you how to cleanse your body fast with juices, vegetables, fresh fruits, herbs, and vitamins, which are instrumental in getting

the colon/bowels, body, and spirit in good working order and maximize your energy level.

This will subsequently begin to yield a substantial amount of weight loss, simply due to proper colon/bowel ELIMINATION.

By following this program, you can be counted as one of the many who has experienced tremendous success in turning your life around by Taking Care of Your Body and "Losing Weight At The Same Time." What have you got to lose, except fatigue and excess weight?

Consider these Principles for Better Health and longer life.

Heredity: These are the traits and characteristics that you have inherited from your parents and grandparents. If your mother or father had heart disease or any other lifelong ailments, then you may have a weakness toward those diseases of ailments as well. If there is a history of a certain disease in your family, you should take extra care of your health regarding that disease. Heredity is something you are born with. However, it is what you do with hereditary inheritance and your eating habits that will determine your overall health.

Diet: It has been said, "You are what you eat." While heredity does play a large role in everyone's health, it is not the only factor. A diet with common sense is essential.

By eating the foods that God has designed for us, we can strengthen the organs in our body and enhance good health. These God given natural foods will cause us to have energy, vigor, and be full of life.

Eat an abundance of herbs, raw and gently cooked vegetables, fruits of all kinds, and raw nuts. By eating the natural food that God has given us, we strengthen the entire body, give nourishment to weak organs, help eliminate waste matter from the body and, most importantly, cleanse and purify the liver and blood. The Bible says: "Herbs were given to man as his food and medicine."

Your Will: Your state of mind is of vital importance. How much do you want to be in good health while maintaining the proper weight? How much do you want to be free of disease, discomfort and pain? You can improve your heredity factor. Eat the proper foods with good old common sense, keep the body clean, and exercise daily. Your good health is a lifelong commitment of your will, your attitude, and your thinking. Always remember, God loves you and He wants you well.

Exercise: Stay active. Look to each day as a day of activity. Take a good long walk for at least 20 minutes three to four times a week. Use your body the way God intended.

Exercise oxygenates the blood and is very important to the body's needs. Regular exercise has been proven to improve spiritual, mental, and physical health. Here's what walking can do for you: Ease aches and pains, help you lose unwanted body fat, and increase your energy immensely.

Walking exerts a force of only one and a half times your weight while keeping the body flexible without subjecting it to too much stress. Walking makes you look better. A vigorous walking program can even help you achieve a shapelier body.

Walking will also help strengthen and tone all of your major body groups in your body, especially the shoulders, arms, back, stomach, legs, and buttocks. It also improves circulation and makes the muscle fibers more flexible.

Walking reduces stress, helps you think faster, and is proven to be a natural tranquilizer by providing some "pondering time" for you to wind down from your daily cares.

Evidence is mounting that regular exercise also stimulates the brain, strengthens the heart, and builds strong bones.

Chapter 2

Let's Get Started

To get maximum results from this program, there are some simple guidelines that you will need to follow. You will need to make some dietary changes to decrease the amounts of toxins you are taking in and to enhance the body's ability to get rid of toxins that already exist.

You will begin by detoxifying the liver. The front line of your defense is your LIVER. The liver has five main functions:

1. It is a major part of your body's immune defense, filtering your blood to remove toxins such as viruses, bacteria, yeast, and other poisonous materials.

2. It stores minerals, vitamins, and carbohydrates.

3. It processes bile, a substance that breaks down fats so that it can be digested.

4. It breaks down and detoxifies hormones, chemicals, toxins, and metabolic waste.

The liver cleanses the body and keeps you well. It has three main ways to detoxify the body:

1. It filters the blood.

2. It secrets bile.

3. It uses a two-step enzyme process of detoxification.

About two quarts of blood are filtered through the liver every minute. When the liver is working properly it is able to filter out 99% of the bacteria and other poisonous toxins from your blood before sending the blood back into circulation.

This program of cleansing and detoxification begins with a diet of supplements you will need to take for a period of three days to two weeks to prepare your body for a juice fast and to restore your body following the fast.

The following dietary guidelines will help cleanse and support your liver before and after the detox fast. To further aid in flushing toxins from your body, you may drink vegetable broth at any time.

To get rid of toxins you must avoid cigarettes, alcohol, drugs, and overeating. Consult your doctor if you are on prescription medications before implementing the program.

Avoid the following foods during the liver detox and juice fasting period:

Refined and processed foods, sugars (including honey and syrup), fast foods, fried foods, wheat and corn products. Limit or abstain from meats. Avoid dairy products, margarine, butter, preserved meats, and processed oils (you may use olive oil).

Choose plenty of the following:

Fruits, vegetables, and vegetable soup. Choose cruciferous vegetables such as cabbage, cauliflower, Brussels sprouts, broccoli, kale, collard greens, turnips, and mustard greens.

Other vegetables to eat often are beets, carrots, and all kinds of beans.

Beverages are essential to the detoxification process. Drink plenty of distilled or spring water.

Drink plenty of fresh vegetable and fruit juices. Drink herbal teas, preferably Green Tea, Chamomile, and Peppermint.

Take a comprehensive multivitamin and one mineral supplement daily – one that contains the Vitamin B series, minerals such as zinc, copper, manganese, selenium, and magnesium. Supplements should be taken also to support and strengthen the liver during the detox period.

Our goal is to eliminate toxins from the liver, cleanse the colon of harmful bacteria, and increase the number of bowel movements (2-3 per day) to promote better health and fitness.

As stated earlier, constipation is part of the price we pay for our unhealthy diet. Normal bowel transit time is twenty to thirty hours. If your diet has plenty of fiber, your stools will be soft, but firm. You should also have two to three bowel movements a day on a regular basis.

Normally, bowel movements should occur twenty to thirty minutes after eating; you should have one after every meal. This may be accomplished by consuming the proper amount of fiber (at least 30-35 grams per day), drinking at least eight (8-ounce) glasses of water daily, and regular exercise.

Fiber acts like a broom, sweeping the colon lining, eliminating the toxins, and binding the toxins in the bile so that they cannot be reabsorbed back into your body through the blood.

Most of the chemicals that are detoxified by the liver are contained in the bile, which is dumped in the intestinal tract.

If your GI Tract doesn't have enough fiber or is constipated, then much of the toxic bile is reabsorbed back into your body. This can lead to a multitude of sicknesses, diseases, and other ailments that can plague you throughout your life.

This is the main reason why eating properly, exercising, and maintaining a positive attitude are extremely important if you are seeking to "Take Care Of Your Body" while "Losing Weight At The Same Time."

Chapter 3
Live a Longer and Healthier Life

You should balance your activities with the proper amount of rest. Some of the leading experts in the field of aging now believe that regular exercise, along with the proper amount of rest, may actually add years to your life. Results from a number of tests indicate that speed and muscular strength of many of the elderly can be extended.

Leading authorities agree that this new data is going to shatter many of the myths about aging, mental and physical performance. The conclusion now is that the performance and ability of the elderly have long been underestimated.

Diet, proper sleep, and exercise, along with rest and relaxation, are all important factors in preserving our bodies.

While your diet is extremely important in obtaining a healthier life style, so is your mental attitude.

Laughter is one of the best things for your mental and physical state. People are naturally attracted to someone who has a good sense of humor. You can develop a good outlook and a good sense of humor by associating with and surrounding yourself with pleasant, happy people.

Recognize that stress is a killer. A life filled with stress can really wreak havoc on your body, causing a number of illnesses such as heart attacks, strokes, asthma, gastric problems, menstrual disorders, ulcerative colitis, angina, irritable colon, increased blood pressure, ulcers, headaches, and many other physical challenges.

There are different types of stress, such as mental, emotional, and physical. Emotional stress seems to take the greatest toll on everyone. All stress is not bad; in fact, life would not be very interesting if it were not met with challenges.

However, too much stress, too often with no effective and appropriate outlet, does not allow the body and soul to recuperate. You might review a typical week to see if you can identify things that might be making you anxious or causing you stress. Once identified, stressors can be attacked and eliminated.

Are you a worrier? Chronic worriers don't have more serious problems than others – they just think they do. Many worriers try to cope by trying not to think about their problems, but this just makes things worse. Doctors say that chronic worriers feel less anxious if they actually spend a half hour each day thinking specifically about their problems.

Get plenty of exercise. People who are physically fit look good and feel good.

A good exercise regimen will lengthen your life, improve your appearance, build your self-confidence, and help delay the aging process. That is why I recommend walking as a simple and effective way to get started with a consistent exercise routine.

Remember that you need to do something physical every day. If you don't use your joints, quite simply they will tighten up with age to create the stopped, bent, and worn out appearance we so often associate with old age. Studies have shown that people with arthritis experience less pain if they continue to keep their joints flexible. As one gets older, the bones tend to get brittle. This is why it is common for senior citizens to break bones, and especially their hips, when they fall.

Eating right, getting proper sleep and learning to relax are all very valuable in maintaining a healthy body and mind. And keep in mind that eating healthy foods and avoiding those high in fats, sodium, and cholesterol will help to decrease your risk of heart disease, high blood pressure, and other associated problems.

Chapter 4

The Positive Weight Loss Approach

Once you have made up your mind to begin "Taking Care Of Your Body," you should make that commitment and go into it with a positive attitude.

We all know that losing weight can be quite a challenge. In fact, for some, it can be downright tough. It takes time, practice and support to change lifetime habits. But it is a process you must learn in order to succeed. You, and you alone, are the one who has the power to lose unwanted pounds.

Think like a winner and not like a loser – remember, emotions are like muscles, the ones you use most grow the strongest. If you always look at the negative side of things, you will become a downbeat and pessimistic person.

Even slightly negative thoughts have a greater impact on you and last longer than powerful positive thoughts.

Negative thinking doesn't do you any good. It just holds you back from accomplishing the things that you want to do. When a negative thought creeps into your mind, replace it by reminding yourself that you are somebody, you have self-worth and you possess unique strengths and talents.

Contemplate what lies ahead of you. Losing weight is not just about diets. It is about a whole new you and the possibility of creating a new life for yourself.

Taking Care of Your Body While "Losing Weight At The Same Time" is a program that will appeal to you in several areas and will teach you the behavioral skills you need to stick with it through the weight loss process.

First, you should look for support among family and friends. It can be an enormous help to discuss obstacles and share skills and tactics with others on the same path. You might look for this support from others you know who are in weight loss programs. You can also seek guidance from someone you know who has lost weight and kept it off.

There are success stories about weight loss all across the country today. Television, newspapers, magazines and tabloids all have multitudes of stories about people who have miraculously lost untold pounds and have kept them off. In all instances they say their mental attitude, as well as their outlook on life, have totally changed, thereby creating a total life change.

Unfortunately, most of these programs were in some ways detrimental to the long-term health of these individuals. This is one of the things that has inspired me to lose weight by "Taking Care Of My Body" and to write this book.

Diets and weight loss programs are more flexible now than they once were, and there are many prepared foods available that have been already portioned out. They are made to look attractive and can be prepared in a matter of minutes. Low-fat, Low-sodium and low-calorie foods are on grocery shelves everywhere.

You will probably need to learn the new and wiser eating skills that are found in this book.

You will want a weight loss regimen that gives you some control and flexibility, rather than imposing just one rigid system.

Keep in mind that every good weight loss program will most likely include some physical exercises.

Look at the exercising aspect of this program as fun and recreation and not as a form of grueling and sweaty work. The fact is, physical fitness is linked inseparably to all personal effectiveness in every field of life, not just weight loss. Anyone willing to take the few simple steps that lie between them and fitness will begin to feel better in a short period of time. The improvement will reflect itself in every facet of your existence.

Doctors now say that walking, which I spoke briefly about earlier, is one of the best exercises. It helps the total circulation throughout the body, thus having a direct effect on your overall feeling of health. There are activities such as aerobics, jogging, swimming, and many other exercises that will benefit you as well. Discuss the options with your doctor and take his/her advice in planning your exercise regimen for this program.

Chapter 5

Where Diets Go Wrong

When we decide that we are heavier that we want to be, we have a natural inclination to eat less food.

We may skip lunch or eat only a tiny amount of our dinner in the hope that if we eat less our body will burn off some of its fat. But that is not necessarily true. Eating less actually can make it more difficult to lost weight.

Keep in mind that the human body took shape millions of years ago and at that time there were no diets. The only low-calorie event in people's lives was starvation. Those who could cope with a temporary lack of food were the ones who survived. Therefore, our bodies have developed this built-in mechanism to help us survive in spite of low food intake.

When researchers compare overweight and thin people, they find that they eat roughly the same number of calories. What makes an overweight person different is the amount of fat that they eat. Thin people tend to eat less fat and more complex carbohydrates, fruits, fish, chicken, and vegetables.

Losing weight is not something one can do overnight, but with the Taking Care of Your Body While "Losing Weight At The Same Time" program, you can come real close to doing just that.

A carefully planned program like this is based simply on common sense and certain dietary guidelines.

Unfortunately, there is a lot of misinformation floating around and lots of desperate people are easily duped and ripped off by some of the other so-called dietary health programs out there.

Every day one can read a magazine or newspaper and see advertisements touting some new product, pill, or patch that will take excess weight off quickly.

Everyone seems to be looking for that "magic" weight loss pill. Millions of Americans are trying to lose weight, spending billions of dollars every year on diet programs and products that sometimes lead to poor health. Often they do lose some weight. But, if you check with the same people five years later, you will find that nearly all have regained whatever weight they have lost. In many cases, they are even more overweight than they were before.

A recent survey was done to try to determine if any commercial diet program could prove long-term success. Not a single program could do so. So rampant has the so-called diet industry become with new products and false claims, that the FDA has now stepped in and started clamping down.

Being seriously overweight can develop into a number of diseases and serious health problems. It is now a known fact that when caloric intake is excessive, some of the excess is frequently saturated fat. The myth is that people get heavy by eating too many calories.

Calories are a consideration, it's true, but overall they are not the cause of obesity. Americans actually take in fewer calories each day than they did at the turn of the century. If calories alone were the reason we become overweight, we should all be thin. But, we are not. Collectively, we are heavier than ever. Partly it is because we are more sedentary now than in past years. But equally as important is the fact that the fat content of the American diet has changed dramatically.

People who diet without exercising often get fatter over time. Although your weight may initially drop while dieting, such weight loss consists mostly of water and muscle. When the weight returns, it comes back as fat.

To avoid the weight gain over time, increase your metabolism by exercising regularly. Select an exercise routine that your physician suggests best fits your body type and physical condition; one that you are totally comfortable with. And remember, walking is one of the best and easiest exercises for strengthening your bones, controlling your weight, and toning your muscles.

In the next few chapters we will be focusing on the way to detoxify your system and begin rebuilding your cells through juicing, vegetable combinations, fish, water, and of course, exercise.

Remember, consistency breeds excellence in any given situation and that this one is no different.

I assure you that if you stay consistent with this new program, not only will you lose weight, but also you will change your life for the better in every area.

Chapter 6

Broth Recipes

These broth recipes are essential to get your body in an optimum position to get healthy. The broths will help to cleanse your body as well as provide the necessary nutrients that are needed on a daily basis for clear thought, energy, and weight loss.

USE STAINLESS STEEL POTS FOR ALL BROTH MIXTURES

Broccoli Broth

Fresh Broccoli

Garlic Cloves (2-3)

Parsley (2-4 Stems) per quart of broth

Braggs Natural Seasoning (for taste)

Cut broccoli into pieces (including the stems). Add water to the pot to accommodate the amount of broccoli used. Add garlic, parsley and Braggs seasoning. Bring to a boil, then lower temperature and simmer for 30-45 minutes. Steam the broccoli (not too mushy). Blend a portion of the cooked broccoli in a blender. Remove the garlic and parsley pieces from the liquid. Pour the blended broccoli into the reserved liquid. Refrigerate until needed. The broth may be reheated in the microwave oven before drinking. Drink as often as desired.

Vegetable Broth

8 medium size carrots

1 medium size beet (include the top)

2 stalks of celery

4 cubed red potatoes (include the skin)

½ bunch of parsley

½ head of cabbage

1 dash cayenne

1 tablespoon of oregano

1 tablespoon of thyme

Braggs Seasoning to desired taste

Bring water to boil, turn temperature down to simmer and add all ingredients except herbs and seasoning. Simmer for 1 hour. During the last 15 minutes add the herbs (oregano, thyme and Braggs Seasoning. After broth is cooled, remove all vegetables and refrigerate broth until needed. The broth may be reheated in the microwave oven before drinking. Drink as often as desired.

High Potassium Broth

½ cup of diced potatoes

1 ½ cup mixed vegetables (such as carrots, broccoli, spinach, celery and peas)

2-½ cup of water

Braggs Seasoning to taste

Combine all ingredients, except seasoning, in pot over medium heat. Cook until vegetables are tender, about 10-12 minutes. Cool vegetables and puree in blender or food processor until very smooth. Pour pureed vegetables into broth and reheat. Season to taste (using Braggs Seasoning). Drink as often as desired.

Corn Broth

6 whole ears of corn (any size)

1 large onion

3 cloves garlic

2 cubed tomatoes

1-tablespoon oregano

Add Braggs Seasoning as needed to taste

Add water up to half of medium stainless steel pot. Scrape the kernels from the corncob. Add kernels and cobs along with remaining ingredients to pot. Simmer on low for 30-45 minutes. Remove some of the corn kernels, cool and blend. Add the remaining cooled ingredients to the blender and blend. When all ingredients are blended, add to liquid they were cooked in. Strain if too thick. Cool and refrigerate until used. May microwave if desired. Also, you may combine any vegetables and herbs of your choice using the cooking instructions above to make your own special broths.

Salads

1. Lettuce (no iceberg)

   Tomatoes

   Cucumbers

   Broccoli

   Carrots (shredded)

2. Cucumbers (sliced – no seeds)

   Tomatoes (halved and sliced)

   Broccoli

   Cauliflower

   Green Onions

3. Spinach (leaves)

   Lettuce (no iceberg)

   Cabbage red/green (shredded)

   Cilantro

   Carrots (shredded)

   Red and green bell pepper (sliced)

Dressing:

   Balsamic Vinegar

   Extra Virgin Olive Oil

   Sprinkle Salt and Pepper

Chapter 7

Vegetable and Fruit Juice Combinations

Here are a series of very powerful and delicious vegetable juice combinations that will boost your energy, detoxify your liver and cleanse your colon for much better bowel elimination. You can make these drinks with any of today's juicers, which may cost from $20 to $200, depending upon the model. Somewhere in the middle of this figure is generally the price range for an excellent and efficient juicer.

It will be worth its weight in diamonds by the time that you get half way through the "Taking Care Of Your Body" program.

Place all ingredients in Juicer at the same time.

#1

2 medium carrots

3 stalks celery

½ large cucumber

¼ bunch parsley

¼ medium beet (with stems)

1 medium apple

#2

2 medium carrots

3 large leaves collard greens

3 stalks celery

¼ bunch parsley

1 medium apple

½ large cucumber

#3

2 handfuls spinach

1 medium apple

1 bunch parsley

2 stalks celery

2 medium carrots

#4

2-½ stalks celery

½ large cucumber

3 medium carrots

½ bunch parsley

2 small apples or 1 large apple

10-15 dark grapes

#5

3 medium carrots

3 stalks celery

1 medium cucumber

#6

3 medium cucumbers

1 clove garlic

2 medium apples

#7

2 tomatoes

2 medium carrots

2 medium cucumbers

2 medium apples

#8

3 leaves collard greens (with stems)

2 medium cucumbers

2 small carrots

1 handful of parsley

1 apple

#9

3 medium carrots

1 handful parsley

1 handful spinach

4 leaves collard greens (with stems)

1 medium to large apple

#10

½ head cabbage

2 medium carrots

1 handful spinach

1 handful parsley

2 medium apples

Fruit Juice Combinations

#1

2 medium apples

2 medium oranges (peeled)

1 small lemon (peeled)

½ bunch dark grapes (20-25 grapes)

#2

2 medium apples

1 pink grapefruit

1 small lemon

¼ melon

#3

4" slice of pineapple

2 medium apples

2 small peaches

1 medium orange

#4

1-cup strawberries

1-cup blackberries

1 cup blue berries

1 pink grapefruit

1 medium apple

#5

2 medium oranges

1 small banana

2 medium apples

1 lemon

#6

1-cup watermelon

1 small banana

2 medium apples

1 lemon

#7

1 grapefruit (peeled)

1 medium orange (peeled)

2 medium apples

#8

Watermelon (with rinds)

10 strawberries

#9

½ melon or cantaloupe

1-cup berries

1 medium apple

#10

2 medium apples

2 large peaches

1 small bunch grapes

Chapter 8

Daily Schedule

The most important thing to remember and adhere to if you want this program to be successful, is to be consistent with your daily schedule.

You don't have to get neurotic about it, but try your best to remain consistent, and if you should happen to get off track, don't get discouraged – it happens to everyone!

Get right back on track with your schedule again and keep on dropping pounds and getting healthier every minute.

Stick with your schedule and by the time you get half way through the "Taking Care Of Your Body" program, you'll be sending me a thank you letter.

Here are some basic steps to a better "You!"

1. Take your HERBS (as directed on package) at least 30 minutes prior to your breakfast (juice). Try to take them around 7:00 a.m. or so, JUICE at 8:00 a.m. (8-12 oz).

2. About 10:00 a.m. drink about 8-10 ounces of BROTH (made from one of the recipes). Also take a multi-vitamin and Systems Strength Recovery Broth at this time. Systems Strength Recovery Broth should be taken once daily (refer to directions on label).

3. For lunch drink 8012 ounces of JUICE or BROTH, along with any fruits or vegetables of your choice. You may have salad (no meat). After eating lunch go walking for 20 minutes.

4. In the afternoon, about 2:30 – 3:30 p.m. drink 8-12 ounces of BROTH.

5. Between 5:30 and 6:00 p.m. take your evening HERBS as directed on label.

6. At 6:30-7:00 p.m. drink 8-12 ounces of JUICE along with any fruits or vegetables of your choice. You may also have salad (no meat). Remember, no iceberg lettuce on any salads.

- The total JUICE and BROTH taken during the day should be between 1-½ pints to 1-½ quarts.

- You may drink HERB TEA and BROTH as desired through the day.

- Drink at least 8 (8 ounce) glasses of water daily.

- If at anytime you become too hungry, eat a small apple, orange, grapefruit or 10-15 dark grapes.

- Try to stay on the JUICES, BROTH, FRUITS and VEGETABLES as many days as you can before introducing solid foods again.

When re-introducing solid foods:

- Continue taking HERBS as directed.

- Breakfast: Drink 8-12 ounces of JUICE at approximately 8:00 a.m.

- For mid-morning snack eat fresh fruit (grapes, apples, oranges) and water/juice/broth/tea as desired.

- Lunch: Eat 3-4 ounces of fish, chicken (white meat), salmon or tuna (meat should be baked, broiled, grilled or poached). In addition, eat as many raw/steamed vegetables or green salad as desired.

- Between 5:30 and 6:00 p.m. take evening HERBS (eat dinner at least 30 minutes after).

- Dinner: Same as lunch. If you have salad for lunch have vegetables for dinner or vice-versa. Have meat from the same meat group as lunch, but different from the meat you had for lunch. Have a glass of water/juice/broth/tea after dinner.

- Evening snack: fresh fruit, vegetables, herbs, tea, water or broth.

- He times listed in this schedule are indicated as guidelines only. They may be easily customized to fit your specific daily routine.

Raspberry Vinaigrette

1-cup water

2 tablespoons honey

1-tablespoon arrowroot (available at health food stores)

½ cup raspberry vinegar

½ tablespoon stone-ground mustard

Combine water, honey and arrowroot in pan over low heat. Stir until mixture thickens. In separate bowl combine vinegar and mustard and mix well. Whisk into honey mixture.

Use 1 tablespoon over salads or vegetables. Place salad or vegetables in a zip lock bag. Close bag and shake to evenly distribute dressing.

Juice Combination

Yields 2 ½ cups (approximately 20 ounces)

2-½ stalks celery

½ large cucumber

3 peeled carrots

10 stems parsley

2 small apples

10-15 dark grapes

You may have fresh fruit, fresh vegetables or sales as desired when hunger takes you over. Limit sale intake.

Be Blessed

The following herbs & seasonings can be purchased at any health food store:

Ultimate Cleanse

Systems Strength Recovery Broth Mix

Braggs Seasoning

Acknowledgments

I wish to acknowledge my indebtedness to the following people:

My three children, for being there, encouraging me along the way. My son Derrick for his untiring enthusiasm, encouragement, and prayers. My son Frederick Jr. and daughter, Tara, for their frequent compliments and prayers, during the down times (they would constantly say, "Mom, you don't need to lose any more weight"). Thanks for being my biggest fans.

My grandsons Derrick II, Dimi II, and Josiah for always being my fans, saying "Grandma you're getting too skinny." Giselle Walsh from Rancho Health Food Store for her excitement each time I visited the store. She would say, "I can't recognize you any more, you look sooooo good!"

My siblings for their encouraging me each time they saw me as the weight just dropped off right before their eyes.

My friend and Sister in the Lord, Dr. Vicki Lee Johnson, who would not allow me not to write this book.

And, last but not least, my Sister/friend Rose Knott and her family. Rose was there **every day**, either by phone or in person. Rose would say, "Girl you can do anything that you set your mind to." "I know you can do this program."

We accomplished our goals together while Taking Care of Our Bodies and "Losing Weight At The Same Time". I love and appreciate each of you.

Important Information

The following was used daily in conjunction with the program

*Ultimate Cleanse Colon Cleanse

*Braggs Seasoning

Daily Multi Vitamin

* May be purchased in most Health Food Stores

Contact Information

We hope you enjoyed this amazing book by

Rita Knott-Woodfin

To order additional copies of this book,

Schedule a speaking engagement,

Or

To Contact

Rita Knott-Woodfin

Write/Call

Vision Keepers Publication

P. O. Box 8212

Ranch Cucamonga, California 91701

951.318.3910

E-mail: visionkeeper2@gmail.com

Facebook

https://www.facebook.com/rita.knottwoodfin

www.ingramcontent.com/pod-product-compliance
Lightning Source LLC
Chambersburg PA
CBHW060220290526
45789CB00003B/1346